Kathleen,

To my friend and mentor,

with gratitude,

Kathleen R. Hopkins

Getting a Grip

By
Kathleen Hopkins

Indo American Books

2261, Ground Floor, Hudson Line, Kingsway Camp, Delhi-110 009
(INDIA) Phone : + 91-011-42870094, E-mail: sales@iabooks.com
Web. : www.iabooks.com

@
2016

Book Team
President : Vijay Sharma
Sr. Vice President : Puneet Singh (London)
Vice President : Kanika Sharma (London)
Pre-Press : P. K. Mishra
Vice-President Marketing : Agnel Henry

I S B N : 93-82661-37-9

Digitally Printed & Published in India with permission from the copyright holder by
Indo American Books
2261, Ground Floor, Hudson Line, Kingsway Camp
Delhi 110009, INDIA. Ph.: 91-011-42870094
Email: sales@iabooks.com
Website: www.iabooks.com

Table of Contents

Foreword

Dr. Hopkins has produced an intriguing book, thus joining other masterful experts in clarifying the importance of handwriting instruction and practice. In opposition to the current trends of promoting screen time and keyboard use by students, educators and parents have overlooked the benefits of handwriting in stimulating several areas of the brain, creating deeper memory pathways, lowering emotional tension, increasing fine-motor coordination, producing fluency, establishing multi-processing efficiency, and clarifying personal thoughts. Dr. Hopkins and I have shared a long-term friendship, as well as professional camaraderie. We shared the benefits of knowing and learning from experts whose lifework was to develop effective strategies in teaching students with learning disabilities. Together, we served in developing NILD, originally called the National Institute for Learning Disabilities and now entitled The National Institute for Learning Development. This agency has trained hundreds of effective therapists who, in turn, have resolved the learning challenges faced by thousands of students. I have been honored to be her colleague and friend. I trust that this publication will accomplish its purpose in awakening parents and professionals to the mandate of handwriting instruction and practice.

Sharon R Berry, PhD
Christian Deaf Fellowship
Birmingham, Alabama

Acknowledgements

I am extremely grateful to my colleagues at NILD who have encouraged me over the past ten years to "Please write this book!" It has gone through many iterations involving piles of data, multiple school visits and interviews with many whom you will find in the text. In short, it has taken on a life of its own and I have needed to exercise the patience to wait for it. (Not one of my strong suits!)

Special thanks go to Susannah Dailey, my daughter and special education teacher par excellence from whom many of these ideas have flowed. She lives the humor and pathos daily as she extends grace to struggling learners.

I am indebted to Tamara Thornton, Yale University Press, whose thorough research of "Handwriting in America" has provided historical documentation for some of the reasons surrounding the current handwriting dilemma in America today. Truly, there is both humor and pathos as we watch the profound changes taking place in literacy. Thank you, Tamara, for your fine contribution.

I received several refusals by publishers who found the book to be a "niche" market, not mainstream, nor relevant for learners today. How sad, America! Then along came a publisher from

India, who loved it and now its message will be shared world-wide. God moves in mysterious ways his wonders to perform.

Special thanks also to my husband, Ralph, whose patience greatly exceeds mine!

Introduction

It is time we began to dive more deeply into both the art and the science of education. Each subject area is woven into another seamlessly as if by an unseen hand. The scarlet thread running through all is the art and science of written expression, our most complex human achievement.

Dr. Hopkins

Chapter 1

I Can't Read German!

James was just shy of his 12th birthday when he was assigned to a special education classroom. Drowning in the details of schoolwork, he preferred to watch his rather beautiful teacher as she moved toward the front of the room. Her hair encircled her head like a halo of light and her stunning dress had amazing designs all over it. He began to count the patterns of dots, or were they ovals? She began to write on the board something that appeared foreign. James' hand shot up. "Miss Dailey, I can't read German".

"James, this is cursive writing", replied his amused teacher. "I know you have not seen this in a while but it is important that we can at least recognize it even if we do not use this kind of writing in our class work. Can anyone help James with decoding the sentence?" A few hands went up.

In truth, cursive writing is rapidly disappearing from schools across the land. James is not alone in his inability to recognize the circular "joined up" letters. It appears to have come from another century and most certainly has little relevance for learners today, particularly those struggling learners who have great enough difficulty mastering simple print. "In an era emphasizing evidence-based instructional practices, it is puzzling why neither handwriting nor spelling is included in the Common Core State Standards for Writing K-5. "Considerable research shows that both handwriting and spelling support the written expression of ideas." (Berninger, V. 2012)

James continued to gaze at the board, then at Miss Dailey. His thoughts rambled as he looked at the rather "cool" writing. He considered the flowing lines and wondered if he could create his own special signature if he could learn this foreign looking script. He made up his mind to ask her about it at the end of the day then spent the rest of the afternoon creating circles and ovals.

At last the school bell ended the day and the classrooms emptied quickly. Miss Dailey had bus duty so was rounding up stray book bags for children who needed special assistance and was barking orders to a few wanderers. Feeling depleted, she looked forward to going home and putting her feet up with a glass of some adult beverage. Inwardly she smiled at James' remark about the German writing. "These kids are so fabulous", she mused. "They never fail to make my day. I cannot imagine teaching students who always know the answers. With my group it is a laugh every minute! How funny that James thought cursive writing was German"!

Just then James came charging at full speed knocking her into an empty wheelchair! "Miss Dailey, I want to learn how to write in that fancy way. Can you teach me? "I would love to, James, but we have no time in the school day for that", Miss Dailey responded with some effort as she climbed out of the wheelchair. Shoulders stooping, James headed to his bus.

By the time students with special needs reach middle school most of them print all their school work. Often the printing is illegible and the effort to wrap untrained fingers around a pen or pencil can be painful.

"Dysgraphia affects up to 30% of US children in third to fifth grades impairing both academic and personal achievement." (Conti, G., 2012)

Because most schools rely heavily on worksheets and varied demands of written expression in the classrooms this difficulty in putting pencil to paper limits the ability to fluently communicate what students really know. Keyboards are often suggested as a helpful alternative. For students like Matt, trying to find the necessary keys to produce the correct spellings of these missed words only lead him into frustration. Miss Dailey had tried that.

James kept thinking about that unusual writing on the board as he rode home. He took out his practice paper of circles and ovals and as the bus bumped along he enjoyed seeing what interesting patterns his pencil made; he was creating something really cool. He couldn't wait to show his mom who was his biggest fan.

Generally, it is mom who supports and encourages students who find school difficult. Despite this nurturing often the tears fall throughout the drills and practices. Parents tend to blame themselves for the endless struggles and long for an end to the torture that looms large each afternoon.

This day, however, James bounded off the bus with his slightly crumpled page of circles and ovals. "Guess what Mom; I saw some writing on the board that looked foreign. Miss Dailey said it was "cursed" or something like that. I asked if she would teach me but she said it would take too much time at school. Can you teach me? Mom agreed to try but only after the homework was finished. As it turned out, two important tests were on the agenda the next day and no time was left.

The ability to write well in a strong hand is only accomplished after much practice. Because fluent script, after learned, flows more easily than print, it requires the cooperation of many cognitive systems. But before a child enters school these fine motor systems are to be trained through play. Old fashioned games such as marbles, jacks, handstands, climbing, etc. require and build digital strength. Toys like building blocks, Lego's, coloring books, throwing and catching balls all equip the hands to write well before students ever put a pencil to paper. Today's students use thumbs and forefingers to sweep across computer screens but the other digits lie mostly dormant. This lack of hand strength translates to a big problem when they must show what they know by writing. The brain and the hand have not been well trained to work together through practice. Thumbs can only do so much alone.(Mangen, 2012)

Personal reflection

Pause a moment and look at your hands. Spread them out in front of you, palms down. Depending on your handedness see if there is a "writing bump" on a finger somewhere. See that as a battle scar. Most teachers today did learn handwriting, the cursive kind, in school and we have a mark to prove it. Now, let's see what you remember. Take a pencil (not pen) and write the letters of the alphabet, both upper and lower case in that cursive alphabet that most likely was above the board for reference in your classroom. Give yourself a grade for remembering.

Chapter 2

The Power of the Hand

James had few friends in school but one was a big guy who liked to arm wrestle the other boys. Tyler was the champ at that, undisputed. He set up matches regularly and James enjoyed trying to beat him. In fact, his right hand was getting stronger as he challenged Tyler to fit in a match most days after lunch. James enjoyed watching the muscle in his arm expand. Miss Dailey observed this particular match with interest. "Finally, something James is really good at", she smiled. "Hey, James, I think I may be able to fit in a handwriting lesson before class begins. You interested?"

James had hoped she might remember. After homework last night he had gone to his room and practiced some more of those circles and ovals. He even launched into creating some new shapes that were even fancier. Smiling, he tried a version of his own name that looked fantastic. He really wanted Miss Dailey to see it.

Older generations regarded cursive writing as an art form, unique to each individual. It allowed freedom of expression and in a special way reflected the personality of the writer. Hand-written diaries and personal notes to friends each contained the essence of the person who wrote them, just as when letters were impressed with the seal of the sender. In our rapidly changing digital culture we have exchanged warmth and personality for a new, faster form of communicating. But, the problem goes much deeper than the resulting shallow relationships.

As James and Miss Dailey enjoyed a few minutes before class began, she looked at his pages of rather unsophisticated script. These were not letters exactly but a good effort to produce his name in joined scrolls. He was obviously very proud of his work "Right, James, I can see you are eager to learn more about this way of communicating". (Oh, my, she thought, how will I ever be able to fit cursive instruction into my very busy day? Seriously, what have I gotten myself into?) James sensed her panic rising and responded. "It's okay, Miss Dailey, I will keep practicing."

During the day this conscientious teacher began observing more carefully the strange ways students were holding their pencils. She grimaced at the labor intensive efforts, tongues extended, brows furrowed, hands cramped and wondered how much their ability to transfer their thoughts to paper was being compromised by their extreme discomfort in the writing process itself. Then she had one of those brainstorms that flew unexpectedly into her lovely head. James noticed her smile and smiled back. His thoughts wandered to admiration again. She was always so kind to him even though his work was often below what he knew was his best. He clenched his fists in frustration. He had become rather proud that he could use either hand to write; not many of his classmates could do that. Recently, though, he had begun using his right hand more since that was the one he sometimes beat Tyler with in hand wrestling. It was definitely becoming stronger.

Miss Dailey pondered. We are supposed to identify a class project and turn it in to the principal next week. What if we somehow worked on this writing business and see if changing to all cursive writing brings our class grades up. It's certainly worth a try. I will need to carve out some precious time in the school day but if these students get as excited as James about learning how to write "German" it may not be too hard to sell. In her characteristic flamboyant way she raised her fist and shouted "Yes! Let's do it! The students looked up and smiled, being used to Miss Dailey's vibrant outbursts. It was part of what made learning fun. This class was about to launch an adventure. James' eyes sparkled with joy.

Despite research from the field of cognitive science that cursive writing plays a strategic role in developing literacy, many schools have traded precious time in the school day for drill and practice of another kind: memorization of facts. Passing the required tests has taken a front row seat relegating learning processes to the back row. Both spelling and handwriting are considered marginal skills today and mostly superfluous to success in this digital age. A sad fallout of this position in the world of education is the report that occupational therapists are seeing more clients than ever before who find handwriting particularly difficult. For students still need to do a great deal of writing in school. Pencil grips have become tortuous defaulting to a "whatever works" method. "For many teachers, having children spend hours copying flowing letters just isn't practical in an era of high stakes standardized testing. Third graders may get 15 minutes of cursive practice a couple times a week and after the fourth grade, it often falls off completely because teachers don't require assignments to be written in cursive." (Hoag, Associated Press, 2012).

No longer considered as one of the three R's, Reading, (w)Riting , and (a)Rithmetic, learning to write by hand is considered irrelevant and time-consuming. Sadly, many educators are not aware that both reading and arithmetic are negatively impacted by the growing weakness of the hand to write. (Grigorenko, 2012).

Skills of keyboarding build very different cognitive systems than writing by hand.   Even very young students are now being required to learn keyboarding skills in kindergarten though their fingers cannot quite stretch across the key monitors.

Personal Reflection

Pause a moment to check your grip. Is your pencil resting comfortably between your thumb and forefinger with your third finger (most likely the one with the bump) supporting the other fingers? It may have been awhile since you wrote in cursive but try a simple sentence. Now write the same sentence in print. What changes do you notice? Most likely you found raising and lowering the pencil while printing was tiring and you may have had to stop and think how to form the cursive letters.

Chapter 3

The Road Less Traveled

On this day James pictured in his mind the great times he used to have in kindergarten. Writing was not such a big deal then. His younger brother brought home all sorts of great art work that James admired. James hoped to become a scientist one day although he had never told anyone that. He supposed that would become a big joke to his fifth-grade classmates since he could barely write his own name. Miss Dailey would not laugh though.

Emerging from his musings, the assignment was to write a paragraph on the science lesson. Today, the students were to use the computer which eliminated the pain of Miss Dailey not being able to read what they wrote but the computer did not help James a bit with gathering and organizing the ideas that he had. Actually, he had lots of ideas but they came into his head like hail falling from the sky and he never had time to collect and express them before they fell to the ground and melted. James hated to disappoint Miss Dailey. She was always so kind, patient and understanding. A lump lodged in his throat as he stared at the keys. Quietly, he pulled out his scrolls and found that a sentence was beginning to form in his mind. With a smile, he pushed aside the computer and wrote it on his paper in beautiful curlicues. He could almost read it and it totally made sense. For the first time in his life James felt hope.

Mastery of script by a child is one of the most important signs of a child's socialization into humanity and its intellectual treasures. Writing is the principal basis for the development of abstract thinking. Writing transforms our cognitive abilities, heightening awareness of the implicit properties of language. Writing shapes thinking. (Grigorenko, 2012)

"When we write, a unique neural circuit is automatically activated. It seems this circuit is contributing in ways we did not realize. Learning, it appears, is made easier. Increased fMRI studies are indicating that when children draw or write freehand they exhibit increased activity in three areas of the brain that are activated in adults when they read and write. By contrast, children who type or trace the letters showed no such effect. (New York Times, 2014). It appears a free hand contributes to cognitive fluency not just in the production of script but in forming ideas that enhance written expression.

Our growing use of screen-based media has strengthened visual-spatial intelligence, which can improve the ability to do jobs that involve keeping track of lots of simultaneous signals, like air traffic control. But that has been accompanied by new weaknesses in higher order cognitive processes, including abstract vocabulary, mindfulness, reflection, inductive problem solving, critical thinking and imagination.

The startling statistics of the college admissions race are reporting that students must find tutors who will help them write their admissions essays. In a recent letter to the Editor of the Virginian Pilot this view was expressed:

"As an educator, I find the elimination of Old Dominion University's writing exam as a requirement for graduation to be troubling news. The fact that many students welcome this decision points to a larger problem within America's schools. From the earliest grades, the focus has become access to information to pass the required tests, with little or no regard for the very important processes of learning.

Handwriting, spelling and grammar are part of a distinct literacy braid that must be continually enhanced and developed at every grade level. Memorization of facts can only prime cognitive systems, not develop them. Dislike of writing, which has reached epidemic proportions has at its roots the failure of teachers across grade levels to weave these important elements into the curriculum. Our focus has been on product, while ignoring the process. It is time to revisit both the art and the science of written expression. Consider the framers of the US Constitution and the Declaration of Independence, who wrote with clarity and skill. It was because they were great thinkers.

Removing a writing essay as a requirement in becoming an educated, literate individual, diminishes us as a nation and will ultimately lead to decreased abilities to solve problems, innovate and graduate. Let's begin again, in kindergarten."

(Hopkins, 2012)

"Handwriting is to written expression as a brush is to a painter" *(Berniger, Handwriting Research Summit, Washington, DC 2012)*

James found himself on a road less traveled. He was learning the love of writing. Indeed, he was discovering a way to become a nuclear scientist. Neither he nor his teachers had any idea that the internet and keyboarding, with all their benefits, had such limitations in the process of developing brains for the high demands of the 21st century.

Miss Dailey passed by James' desk and smiled. In legible cursive he had written

"When I see a molecule inside I can understand the reason why it holds together".

Miss Dailey had tears in her eyes.

Personal Reflection

Take a note card and write a message to a friend. By now, as an educated adult, you have most likely mastered the art of writing. Think about how your handwriting has changed over the years. If you have some written exhibits of 10 or 20 years ago, take a look at them. What message do you take away? There are many possible explanations for the changes you may have noticed. The point is, our handwriting skills are modifiable.

Chapter 4

A Plan Unfolds

James continued his pursuit of literacy throughout the year with Miss Dailey. His attempts at fluent handwriting became more legible and he found his grades improving. Others teased him a bit about his floral designs but he was beginning to hold his own with the arm wrestling so they did not push him too far. He continued, despite lack of instruction, to turn in all assignments with the unique script he had created. Fortunately, Miss Dailey had no difficulty reading it.

Unfortunately, the school principal did not accept Miss Dailey's request to conduct a handwriting study with the fifth-grade class. Too much was at stake with the high profile proficiency testing and handwriting instruction would take far too much precious time out of the school day.

James' brother, Kyle, was in kindergarten and he was very interested in trying to mimic James' letters. Miss Dailey was having lunch with the Kindergarten teacher sharing her disappointment regarding her proposed project when Miss Finch began to warble like a bird! "Kyle has been showing me some of his brother's art work. He wants to try it. I have been very frustrated trying to teach keyboarding to my five year olds. Do you think maybe the administration would agree to let us do an after school handwriting club?"

Miss Dailey broke out in high fives even running toward her buddy, the janitor, with one. The seed was planted and the project began to take on a life of its own. That evening as she drove home, Miss Dailey planned a special meal for her family. Skylights were opening and she sensed fresh joy for an amazing plan that was about to unfold.

As Miss Dailey and Miss Wren surveyed the kindergarten classroom they realized that, interestingly, old fashioned chalk boards still hung on the walls. The children used them during break times to draw pictures with different colored chalk. Other classrooms had been gradually trading chalkboards for the cleaner whiteboards. Some even had smart boards! Miss Dailey noticed how the boards in the kindergarten class seemed less of an eyesore than the smeared whiteboards. New dustless chalk prevented white speckles on the rail and when these boards were clean they looked very inviting. Miss Dailey picked up a piece of chalk and wrote her name with a flourish! My, it took her back a few years! This classroom even had a sandbox, messy but marvelous for sending important signals to the developing brains of these young learners. Light bulbs of excitement flashed in both their pretty heads! "Let's begin with the little ones and let James be a helper in this project!"

Both were veteran teachers, well respected for their giftedness and innovation in the classroom. Other teachers understood that handwriting was a dying art, more or less relegated to antiquity. But some wondered if it was destroying important literacy skills with its demise. What about the literacy braid heralded by fMRI studies which highlighted that marvelous three-strand brain circuitry between spelling, reading and writing? Did the loss of one of these strands jeopardize the other two?

These two veteran teachers began to connect some dots. They talked well into the afternoon after the buses left. From kindergarten to fifth grade the ability to write was deteriorating in all students, not just the less able ones. Most upper classrooms encouraged use of the keyboard to ease the frustration of gripping a pencil and trying to produce ideas. In truth, that did not seem to be working well. Bottom line: students hated to write. So a plan was born.

Armed with the latest information from the field of cognitive science, Miss Dailey and Miss Finch approached the principal with their proposal.

A strong connection exists between fine-motor skills and the development of executive functioning, an important skill need for abstract thinking and written expression. Early handwriting could enhance inhibitory control (that ability to wait until another better idea comes to mind). This ability is a life skill that leads to improved reading and math skills. Science is discovering important relationships between fine motor control and visual-motor integration in such subjects as spelling, reading and written expression. Studies have shown that those who actually wrote letters on paper were better able to recognize and reproduce them from their interior (cognitive) model. The relationship to success in mathematics is a fairly recent finding. Since math has its own distinct language it also relies upon fluid and adaptable thinking.(Grigorenko, 2012)

Indeed, these are scientific words that many teachers tend to dismiss. What is this "brain science" all about anyway? Sadly, the field of cognitive science and the field of education have never stood further apart. Following the "Decade of the Brain" in the 1990's many "brain-based" programs flooded the educational marketplace creating confusion and caution. We are now in a more sophisticated place with improved technology and replicated studies. Still, there remains a great gulf between the two fields, with Schools of Education giving barely a nod to the Schools of Cognitive Science. The greatest casualty of this lack of shared of communication is found in the increasing numbers of third graders who are unable to read in the most advanced country in the world. (Hooper, Handwriting Summit, Washington, DC, 2015)

At the turn of the 20th century, teachers in American schools predicted illiteracy would be eradicated within 10 years. They had sharp tools in the late 1800's and an intuitive sense that the Three R's were sufficiently powerful to train both the mind and the hand to read, spell and write. Teachers in Schools of Education had rigorous instruction in the known sciences of language such as morphology, syllabication and grammatical structures. Students did not use worksheets, they copied their assignments with a clear hand into a composition book.

Today, we have traded hands for thumbs.

Miss Dailey and Miss Wren were about to build a bridge.

Personal Reflection

Consider the way your children write. Are they good at it? Do they like to write? How much time are they spending on a computer as opposed to freehand writing or drawing? Now consider their spelling abilities. When they write their spelling words (if they do) in order to remember them, do they print the words or use cursive? Have you wondered whether there may be a connection between fluent writing and spelling abilities? Now think of five rather complex words (three syllables or more) and write them in cursive in your preferred way. Then print them or type them into your computer. Consider the differences.

When we speak to friends about their handwriting it is not long before we hear the word "ashamed" Try asking a colleague this question.

Chapter 5

The Pen is Mightier than the Keyboard

While the two determined teachers continued gathering data to present their case for support to the principal (they were both schooled in the courts of law having personal experience of such things), James found himself on a rainy weekend perusing his grandmother's attic and suddenly made an historic find!

He had often played in this attic, loving the smell of the mysterious old things. This day he found a box that he had not seen before. It looked like just a lot of old papers, but as James examined them more closely he noticed it was a hand-written document. And there was his grandmother's name, right on the front. As he began to decode the rounded script (he was becoming quite good at this now), he discovered it was something called a dissertation, pages and pages of this awesome cursive script, back to front. Whole sections had been erased and then rewritten as it was originally written in pencil. James tried to imagine the ideas flowing from his grandmother's head onto the paper. He found he was actually able to read it, though some of the words did begin to resemble German.

He carried the box carefully down from the attic.

As Miss Dailey and Miss Finch sat down with the principal, Miss O'Sullivan, they found her quite stern and a bit pre-occupied with piles of paper scattered over her desk. Miss Dailey, extremely OCD, found the mess to be quite appalling, but she smiled, trying not to make eye contact. Miss Finch began again to warble. As a kindergarten teacher this was one of her strong tools. She smiled warmly at the rather disheveled principal and launched full speed into the idea of forming a handwriting club. The last words they remembered hearing as they were escorted out of the room were, "So long as you maintain your fidelity to the standards of testing".

Finch and Dailey had chosen the perfect time to launch the project! James would be so pleased! As they skipped through the hall together they had a sense of adventure a bit like zip lining without the net. Miss Dailey took the hands of her favorite student, and wheeled her around in her wheelchair. Sarah smiled. How she loved Miss Dailey's outbursts. Meanwhile James was on his own attic adventure. After showing his grandmother the box, she smiled and said, "Yes, James, this is my work. I still love to write in cursive. I find my ideas come to me more quickly. There is something else in the attic I would like you to see." Together they climbed the stairs.

Another amazing discovery awaited him. Grandmother unwrapped some large laminated cards that were called Rhythmic Writing. They showed in a very sensible way how smoothly and accurately specific strokes became the letters of the alphabet, rather like a puzzle fits together. James was elated. He thought of Miss Dailey and how pleased she would be to know that he was becoming a real fan of this writing business and these must be really valuable because they had chalk dust all over them.

James could not remember being so excited about learning! He decided to bring these cards to show Miss Dailey. He had also found in the attic a top hat and a long stick, certainly not belonging to grandmother! Standing with the stick extended he imagined being in a circus crying "Ladies and gentlemen" to a rapt audience. He believed he could illustrate how these letters on the historic laminated cards flowed together to make a word. It was almost like magic.

As quick as a flash a new idea popped up. He could actually picture himself in front of a group of kindergarten students instructing them in the art of handwriting! Wouldn't Miss Dailey be pleased!

Studies have been conducted revealing that second, fourth and sixth grade children with and without handwriting disabilities were able to write both more and faster when using a pen rather than a keyboard to compose essays.

Children in kindergarten are still required to do many fine-motor tasks with pencil and paper. By fourth grade 85% of class work requires the use of paper and pencil. Many studies have indicated that handwriting readiness in the early grades is associated with both reading and math abilities in later grades. (Berninger, Handwriting Research Summit, Washington, DC, 2012). Yet writing has become painful and disliked by many children because they have not been trained how to do it easily.

Letter writing by hand requires serial component strokes and has its own unique written language register in the brain that is distinct from the circuitry required for reading or oral language. Writing is more complex than reading because it places more demands on cognitive functions. The establishment of brain circuitry is uniquely fused through handwriting. This primes cognitive circuitry to be prepared for higher-level planning. The highest level of cognitive interaction, studies are showing, is written expression. In contrast, keyboarding requires far simpler motor-memory.(Conti, 2012)

Personal Reflection

Now let's do another interesting activity. Select a writing instrument, preferably a sharpened pencil and a piece of unlined paper and write your full name with your eyes closed. Surprised? Now, write it again this time with your eyes open. If these two signatures look similar, it means the memory of the letters is well stored in your brain. Now try the same activity with print. Draw your own conclusions. Do you have copies of personal letters written by hand stored away somewhere? Can you imagine saving email messages in the same way?

Chapter 6

A Foundation is Laid

It was winter and snow covered the ground. James liked these days when he could conduct writing experiments at home. Wrapping his hands around a new quill pen, he dunked it in the inkwell and loaded the black ink without spilling a drop. How cool was it that his great-grandparents had written with inkwells in their desks! Today, he was ready to compose his first paragraph with this new tool.

He thought it would be a good idea to do some warm up strokes so carefully he wrote the upper and lower case letters of the alphabet. He would not have known what they looked like if he had not found the amazing pages of Rhythmic Writing. The first attempt was a bit wobbly, so he tried again, this time at the chalkboard, which his mom had given him as a special gift. The beautiful letters flowed from the chalk in the holder onto the board. He found it helpful to say the names of the strokes as he went along, "over, back, around." They looked fantastic! Back to the inkwell...

The resistance of chalk sliding along a board sends a strong sensory signal to the brain's cognitive circuits. This is in contrast to the smooth writing on a paper or whiteboard which sends no signals. It is this neural feedback that primes the brain to enable the hand to write so that the brain itself can be freed to think about what to write, not how.(Zimmerman,1976)

All afternoon James created some brilliant ink monograms of his favorite letters. He was totally using his right hand and the ink was not even blotching. He was so surprised that he actually enjoyed something he used to hate. His thoughts went to Miss Dailey. Then he had an idea. He would take a phone photo of his monograms and email it to Miss Dailey. He could picture her smile.

James managed to become quite good at each of the letters and their component parts (motifs) on page one. Just then Kyle walked in his room, bored with yet another snow day.

"Hey, James, what are you doing?"

"Creating cool stuff", James replied. Then he had an amazing thought. "Let's see if I can teach Kyle how to write like this."

Donning his top hat and grabbing his stick James positioned himself before the board as Miss Dailey did and pointed to the capital letter A written in smooth cursive. Kyle knew his alphabet but was not familiar with this shape. Suddenly he cried out, "That is an A, I have seen it written like that on my "Angry Birds" video!

"Perfect, Kyle, sit in that chair over there, I want to teach you a lesson".

At the end of this snow day, James had managed to train Kyle in how to write the first three letters of the alphabet, upper and lower case. Kyle ran downstairs to show his mom who smiled for the first time that day. (Moms so love snow days!)

Standing before a chalkboard also works on the vestibular (balance) and proprioceptive (body position) systems. Crossing the midline activates communication between both hemispheres and increases the brain's ability to specialize in what it does best. Zimmerman, (1985)

Some educators have compared the act of printing words as "dot to dot" painting by numbers, and in contrast, cursive writing as the rhythmic brush strokes of a true artist. It has also been noted that when children are exposed to cursive writing, the act of physically gripping a pen or pencil correctly helps overcome their motor challenges. In addition, smooth, automatic cursive script activates parts of the brain that lead to increased language fluency.

According to Mangen and Velay (2012) "Writing is an immensely important and equally complex and sophisticated human skill commonly ascribed a fundamental role in children's cognitive and language development and a milestone on the path to literacy." (p 386) Furthermore, Singer & Singer (2005) affirm that "Any theory of human intelligence which ignores the interdependence of hand and brain function is grossly misleading."

Even more amazing is that science confirms the emergence of a mathematical mind space that enables written literacy. As students mature, transcription becomes more fluent and automatic allowing more cognitive space for text as well as generation of problem solving. High level scientific understanding may well be enriched through the construction of such cognitive space through the dual action of the hand and brain.

Of course, James was not aware of these recently understood brain changes, only that he was very excited to finally be learning to write. He decided to end this great day by writing a letter in cursive to his favorite teacher. It was his sincere desire to become a scientist one day and he wanted Miss Dailey to know that. His strong right arm punched the air, "Yes!"

Chapter 7

The Letter

Dear Miss Dailey:

This is the first letter I have ever written to anyone. I wanted you to see what I have been practicing. I also have a secret that I want to tell you. I have always wanted to become a scientist. I know you will not laugh at me but the other kids in my class might. Please don't tell them.

I have a new quill that I am using for this letter. When I write now I can think better. I can understand how and why the ink flows into and out of my pen. And my sentences are longer. Thank you for believing in me.

Your student,

James

The letter arrived on Miss Dailey's desk as she was monitoring the hall. On the first day back from a long snow break, she was not looking forward to the catching up process. It was her job this morning to chase children who had dropped boots and gloves. Three successive snow days would likely set her children back a month. The amount of re-teaching and intensive drill that it would take to get them on track began to diminish her joy. The first child in the room had dropped her lunch box and yoghurt splattered everywhere. Unfortunately, her pal, the janitor, was nowhere to be found.

Then she saw James, smiling from his seat. "I think I can help with that, Miss Dailey." "How kind, James", she replied. I have a pile of boots and gloves to take to the lost and found."

It was lunchtime before Miss Dailey noticed the letter. She did not recognize the fine ornate script but supposed that it was from a parent explaining why, after three days, the homework was not done. The final quarter of the year had begun badly. She felt a headache coming on and the day was only half over. Then she decided to try to settle everyone down by playing Beethoven. The CD was soothing. She picked up the letter.

James was watching as she opened it but was not at all prepared for the effect it would have. Miss Dailey looked at it for a long time. Then she reached into her drawer and pulled out a plate of homemade cookies. James thought, "She is pretty and she can cook too?"

Pushing back her chair Miss Dailey rose slowly to face the class.

In quiet but strong words she announced, "We have a scholar in our class today." The students looked all around and waited. Beethoven played on. One student raised a hand. "Miss Dailey, what is a scholar?

"It is some one who loves to learn. Does that apply to any of you in here?" The class was used to Miss Dailey's strange and funny ways so they began to giggle, waiting for the answer.

Slowly a couple hands went up. Then suddenly every hand was up, but one.

Miss Dailey, wearing James' favorite dress with the ovals, walked with her plate of cookies straight to James' desk. His face was turning red and he wished he could disappear. The giggling stopped.

Miss Dailey continued, "A scholar is also a strong person who can win at arm wrestling and not be proud. Or someone who does lots of homework when it has not been assigned. Or a person who is willing to help clean the floor without being asked. Or one who can learn how to write in cursive just because he wants to.   All eyes turned to James and Miss Dailey handed out her homemade cookies still a bit warm from the oven. They all ate quietly. Beethoven played on and James beamed.

Personal Reflection

When was the last time you wrote a handwritten note? Did you mail it or hand deliver it? Consider why you decided to write it by hand rather than email it. Then decide why you did not send it electronically. Make some observations regarding our culture. Also make some observations as to how the person responded to receiving the written note

Chapter 8

Interesting Coincidences

One improvement Miss Dailey was beginning to notice was the increase in James' spelling grades. Also, he was becoming very proficient using his right hand to do all his schoolwork, explaining to Miss Dailey that words seemed to flow easily from his hand to the paper. It helped that he had been practicing the correct way to make the letters, but Miss Dailey was amazed that reading abilities were also skyrocketing. His title of scholar was becoming a self-fulfilling prophecy. No one made fun of him anymore, especially since he had become "famous" as the "Teacher" for the after school handwriting club.

The club was open to five and six year olds who wanted to learn to write in this great new way. As James stood in front of the eager learners complete with hat and pointer, he noticed that Miss Dailey and Miss Finch beamed at him. They had spent considerable time after school with James until they were certain that he was following the method of Rhythmic Writing on the charts. Today was his debut. "Okay, class, let's begin with the cursive letter A!

Miss Dailey and Miss Finch circled the room checking for correct pencil grip and writing posture. The students were quietly concentrating. Then came the fun part. James would call up one student at a time to write a letter on the board. Eventually, they would join letters into three and four letter words. James could not contain his joy.

After school he spent extra time with the science books he had checked out of the library. He was interested in nuclear science but rocket science held special motivation. He had heard that it might be possible in his lifetime to travel to Mars! Wow, now that would be a trip! But even more exciting would be to actually become an astronaut. One book James selected had drawings of the thrust engines. The designs were fascinating and the intricate connections of the these engines excited his imagination. After studying them for awhile, he found he could reproduce these designs from memory. At times, James wondered why his classmates were not as excited about learning as he was.

James continued to apply himself to the rigorous fifth grade curriculum. He did all his work in cursive now and was clearly the new champion of hand-wrestling. Tyler acknowledged his supremacy with a pat on the back. The icing on the cake was winning the class spelling bee! Could it get any better than this? James took his very first trophy home to his Mom, his constant cheerleader.

Writing is the principal basis for the development of abstract thinking. It heightens the writer's awareness of the implicit properties of language. Writing is not the opposite of reading. Writing requires much more cognitive involvement, particularly the neural networking within working memory.(Grigorenko,2012)

Functional MRI studies have shown that when children draw a letter freehand they exhibit increased activity in three areas of the brain that are activated by adults when they read or write. For those who like to get their heads around specific scientific terms these are known as the left fusiform gyrus, the inferior frontal gyrus and the posterior parietal cortex. By contrast, children who typed or traced the letter showed no such effect.

Researchers have begun to study the comparative quality of the ideas of students who write by hand and those who use the keyboard. Findings have supported that when children compose text by hand they not only consistently produce more words more quickly than on the keyboard, but also express more ideas.

Clear differences now appear between printing and cursive writing in terms of facility of writing, idea generation and number of words produced, a distinction of particular importance as the teaching of cursive disappears across the curriculum.

Studies of high school and adult learners demonstrate that the notes they take from lectures on a keyboard are more difficult to decipher afterwards. Increasing evidence exists to show that taking lecture notes by hand, in established cursive, allows a student to process and reframe the lecture's content more easily than when taking notes on a keyboard.

According to Rose (2004), reading difficulties may relate directly to inadequate printing practice in kindergarten and first grade. Historically, many authorities on the subject of literacy instruction have stressed the importance of adequate practice in printing alphabet letters. Fabius Quintilianius (AD35-98) wrote that in regard to becoming literate, "Too slow a hand impedes the mind". It can be assumed that continued writing in the upper grades keeps literacy fluid and strong.

Miss Dailey approached James in the hall after school. "Hey, I was watching you take notes during the science lesson today.

Could I take a look at them?" "Sure," said James, pulling them out of his backpack. "I thought they might help me with the big test tomorrow. I found it easy to listen and write at the same time. I have never been able to do that before, but today the words just flowed right out of my pencil." Miss Dailey smiled, "You managed to do some underlining too and captured all the key points. Way to go "Scholar."

Skipping down the hall Miss Dailey felt as though she had a gold coin in her pocket. Heading the opposite way to meet his mom, James seems to be walking on clouds!

For centuries handwriting has been an art. To a growing number of young people it has become a mystery. An 18 year old freshman signed her name on a college entrance exam in all printed capital letters. She was unable to produce a proper signature so was denied admission. The news media reported that several in the group desiring admission had forgotten how to write in cursive.

Children today who do not learn the skill of handwriting, like generations before them, may be missing out on an important developmental process. Compared to using two hands to type out letters on a keyboard, writing with one dominant hand uses more complex brain power. Writing by hand is more complicated because it integrates three brain processes. (Berniger, 2012)

Visual: seeing what is on the paper in front of you,

Motor: using your fine motor skills to put the pen to paper and write words receiving physical feedback

Cognitive: remembering the shapes of the letters, their flow that enables correct spelling and greater encryption of content into memory.

Personal Reflection

Let's do an interesting experiment. Using your non-dominant hand write out the following sentence that uses all letters of the alphabet:

The quick brown fox jumped over the lazy dogs.

Now, say the sentence once to yourself, then write it without looking again using your dominant hand. What can you deduce from your efforts? Does it occur to you that an untrained hand would find writing by hand quite difficult?

Chapter 9

The Reading Connection

The Writing Club was going so well, James found himself helping "his students" learn to read with the rhyming words they wrote on the board. They wrote them in cursive so they could see it was a whole word rather than individual letters. James could barely move his stick fast enough for the group to say the words they had written. After every correct sequence, he would tip his hat and bow! What a cool after school job! Miss Dailey and Miss Finch, guardians of the project, clapped in wonder and the 20 students became better readers, writers and spellers as the weeks went by. But no one could measure the fun they were having.

Spring arrived and the data gathering began. To the surprise of many, those in the "Club" surpassed all expectations. Miss Dailey was the happiest of all. However, she had reached a point in the school year that she always dreaded, having to say goodbye to her students who were going on to middle school. She would most likely never see them again.

But a new seed was germinating.

James suddenly had many friends. Some had come into the Handwriting Club mostly out of curiosity and because James put on such a show. The whole school was talking about it. Parents of the children in the Club saw the difference in their abilities to write and in their confidence to try new things. Reading, writing and even math improved. They petitioned the school to continue the Club next year as their children went into first grade but James would not be there.

Taking advantage of some down time Miss Dailey and Miss Wren went out for coffee. Caffeine always helped solved problems such as James' absence. As they sat back in their cozy chairs sipping their coffee they decided to visit James' grandmother. After all, she had the tools that the Club used and might be willing to share them. This day both right hands went up, "Yes!" The expresso had worked! They soon found that the treasures they were seeking had a rich and vibrant history, beyond a grandmother's attic. As they met with James' grandmother, she revealed the story.

"Actually the beginnings of Rhythmic Writing can be traced back to Drs Archie Silver and Rosa Hagin (1969) at New York University Medical Center in the late 1960's. Deborah Zimmerman, a nurse/educator, had been referred to the university by Dr. June Orton, wife of Dr. Samuel Orton, an important pioneer in the field of dyslexia research and developer of the Orton-Gillingham strategies. Deborah hoped that this method of cognitive stimulation, Rhythmic Writing on a chalkboard, might lead to reading improvement. It was a bold and not necessarily popular idea.

In those days, students with learning challenges often had problems not only with reading but also with writing and spelling.

There seemed to be a strong connection between these three important literacy skills. Inability to read, write or spell often led students to default to printing because the cursive writing process was just too difficult.

This, in itself, gave Deborah the insight that training the hand to write well through using a chalk holder, standing at a chalkboard, might stimulate the brain systems related to literacy to become more efficient. Perhaps, she thought, reading, writing and spelling are linked in some way. So she threw all her 97 pounds into a bold new venture.

The grandmother paused and smiled. She sipped her tea and continued,

"You know, Deborah Zimmerman was a woman ahead of her time. As a nurse, she believed brain systems of processing and memory that were weak could be strengthened through exercise and practice. This activity of standing before a chalkboard seemed very odd to educators who would often snort in her direction, saying, "What are you trying to do, change the brain? Impossible! Just accommodate the students' weaknesses."

Deborah's response was simply, "Through the careful analysis of cognitive scientists, it is generally recognized that the brain is an open system, able to change and be changed throughout a lifetime." Zimmerman, 1976

Miss Dailey and Miss Wren were on the edge of their chairs.

Miss Dailey exclaimed, "I knew that in my heart. I have wondered why we just try to make work easier for these students who struggle with literacy. Actually, I raise the bar higher than anyone else does and because my students trust me, they climb those mountains!

Miss Wren was now misty-eyed remembering that she had the privilege of working with five year olds, the youngest ones, right off the bus! Quietly, she mused, "The younger the brain, the easier it is to strengthen those systems. But how do we know where to begin?"

It seemed James' grandmother had the answer to that question, too. She replied,

"A program called "Search and Teach", a scanning intervention for kindergarten classrooms. It was developed by Dr. Rosa Hagin right there in New York Bellevue Center. Through this national award-winning program, all students in the kindergarten class are given a score for potential vulnerabilities that may lead to learning failure. This screening does not measure intelligence but identifies weak or vulnerable areas in a child's performance that could become precursors of later learning difficulties. Yes, Dr. Rosa Hagin was ahead of her time too." (Haqin, R, Silver, A, 2005)

Miss Dailey and Miss Wren could barely contain the joy! They could envision another visit to the principal with a new and revised plan. What an afternoon this had been!

The laminated pages related to Rhythmic Writing continue to be used today by thousands of students who receive assistance for learning problems and find their way to universities and challenging careers, some as astronauts!

Indeed, these students who formerly found learning so very difficult, discovered that they no longer qualified for the category of learning disability that once labeled them. Writing extraordinary admission essays, these highly literate individuals have mastered the skill of communicating their knowledge in cursive, in print, or on the keyboard. Dreams barely imagined have become realities.

Personal Reflection

It is time to try some free writing. As adults, we have most likely defaulted to using only the keyboard or printing our grocery lists. Think of a short paragraph with a surprise ending. Think first, then write in your best cursive. How did that work out for you?

Chapter 10

New Horizons

James had very mixed emotions this last week of school. With his elementary years now almost history, he found himself gazing again in wonder at Miss Dailey. What a cool teacher she has been, never giving up on him, always believing he was a scholar. He hoped the middle school teachers would understand him as she did. Not much chance of that. He remembered he would have at least five teachers and be running to find his next class. He would have to make a model of the hallway and scope out the floor plan. James was becoming very clever at drawing both designs and concepts. He saw them in his head before they made it to the paper.

The patterns on Miss Dailey's dress suddenly came into focus.

"Wait", he muttered, "was that pattern the outline of a fuselage I was reading about in my new book on how to build your own rocket launcher?" The form came easily into his mind, in fact, he pulled out a paper and began sketching. Miss Dailey smiled her glorious smile as she wished all of them a wonderful summer. James lifted his hand for a high five as he passed through the door. Both he and Miss Dailey knew a most promising adventure awaited, not just for James, but for her, as well.

Seeds had been planted firmly in the minds and hearts of both teachers. They had just heard the news that a new principal would be joining the school, giving fresh hope for the changes they were now envisioning for the kindergarten classes. They had placed some ideas on paper since their visit with James' grandmother. A summer workshop was planned and they would ask for permission to make a presentation. The warbling became spontaneous! New year, fresh joy.

Written language seems to be a problem-solving process in which writers attempt to produce a visible, legible and understandable product that emphasizes their declarative knowledge. Components of writing, that is, handwriting, spelling and composition, require simultaneous use of both motor and cognitive processes. As students mature, transcription becomes more fluent and automatic, freeing more cognitive space for coherent, systematic text generation. (Grigorenko, 2012)

After grade 4, good writers should have fluent handwriting skills if they have been carefully trained in the process through the early years. Working memory, holding their knowledge, has become more automatic and because they do not have to stop to recall how a letter is formed, they are free to consider what to write rather than how.

Personal Reflection

One of the most satisfying adult activities is to journal life experiences. The clean smell of the pages, the entries that mark life's passages , and the thought that future generations of your family may know you through your reflections is a worthy pursuit. Why not begin yours today?

Chapter 11

The Shallows

James also had developed a very coordinated hand and thumb action that had been trained how to use the keyboard and could quickly locate and produce information on the computer. In fact, when keyboarding was taught the last semester in Miss Dailey's class he seemed to learn it more easily than his peers. But then these students were not really interested in writing at all. All his fifth grade projects had been done really well using the information he had researched himself. He was quick to come up with Google keywords and even asked Siri as needed. Yes, the computer was a great tool but it was not his master. He wondered why Tyler, his friend and arm wrestling partner, was on his computer all the time. Moving on to middle school was an awesome adventure!

Creating his own special script came in really handy when he met a new girl at middle school. For this occasion, a personal note had to be cool and legible. He practiced two or three versions at home sending Kyle, his younger brother, out of his room several times.

He considered leaving the note on her desk unsigned and see if she could guess who sent it, but that was risky. She might not have noticed him at all and think it was someone else. No, he would sign it and let the chips fall where they may. He was definitely enjoying this new school. He had made lots of friends and his teachers appreciated his enthusiasm. None of them was as great as Miss Dailey though. He wondered how the new Writers Club was doing.

To James' great delight the first science project would be to design a rocket launcher and the class was going to work in groups. Elise had found the note just as she learned they would be in the same group together. Shyly she said, "Thank you for the note. Can you help me read it? I never learned cursive." A new adventure, rather like white water rafting, was about to begin! James sensed the rush as he responded, "I can help with that!"

Most teachers would agree that having access to a computer and all of its possibilities is probably the most significant accommodation a student with dyslexia can leverage to improve academic performance. But is it? The question to be asked is "Do we accommodate vulnerable cognitive functions or is it possible to strengthen them?"

Most people know that the brain is in charge of guiding a pencil to make letters, words and sentences. Guiding a pencil is a bit like driving a car or a school bus. But many people do not know that the brain has two different drivers for the pencil. One is the eyes, the other is muscle memory. It takes much practice to maneuver a school bus around turns and through narrow roads. Learning to write also requires the right kind of practice. So does keyboarding. Which is better and why?

Because we usually write with a pencil on lined paper our brains typically assign the task of "driving" to the eyes at first. It takes time to get the muscle memory into the driver's seat to produce thoughts on paper. When you know the way you can get there more quickly.

Keyboarding requires different skills. Tips of fingers from both hands create a motor memory but do little to improve spelling or generation of new vocabulary. Keyboarding was originally designed for secretaries to transcribe what was being said or had already been written. It was a step up from the Morse Code or Shorthand. It seems reasonable to assume that moving young children onto the keyboard before they learn to write with paper and pencil may well compromise emerging literacy skills. Not to mention the third grader with dyslexia who is struggling to produce words he cannot yet read or spell.

Personal Reflection

How many students do you know who are currently struggling with written expression? Check to see if they are being encouraged to use the computer to write their papers and if that is helping them. Then ask if they like to write by hand. If the answer is "No, because it is too hard" there may be some evidence that they are also poor spellers and reluctant readers with a diagnosis of dyslexia …for which computers can never be the cure. Chalk on a board is an amazing remedy.

Chapter 12

The Rapids

After English class that day James asked Elise if he could walk her home. It was great that he could walk to middle school now and did not have to ride the bus. Turned out she lived just one street away from his house. He found it easier than he thought to talk to her. She was really nice, reminding him a bit of Miss Dailey. Elise thanked him again for the note and asked if he could please read it to her. Her face turned pink. James' did too but he smiled as he nodded, "Yes."

The inability to understand messages from peers has taken on new ramifications in our rapidly changing digital world. The new language of texting eludes some students who are unable to decode the abbreviations that fly furiously onto phones and computer screens. Social gatherings typically involve silent communication even though friends are face to face. A single mis-interpretation can mean a slower student becomes "unfriended." Far worse is the impersonal nature of these various correspondences that require rapid responses and result in shallow relationships.

Handwriting is less important in our lives than it has ever been. One in three students and adults surveyed said they had not written anything by hand for at least six months. Two out of three said that the last thing they wrote was for their eyes only, a hastily scribbled note or a shopping reminder. Does it matter? Things change, after all. But wait, consider a handwritten letter from a soldier on the front. The personal touch somehow does not transmit electronically (Hensher, The missing Link, WSJ, 12/ 30/12)

James invited Elise to sit on his front step so he could read her the note. He had spent some time writing it in his best cursive so there were a few flourishes here and there. He had also carefully checked his spelling.

Dear Elise,

I hope I spelled your name right. I have never known anyone who had such a pretty name. I would like to be your friend but I do not have a cell phone. Could we write notes instead?

Your friend (hopefully),
James

Elise blushed a brighter shade of pink and flashed that winning smile again. She reminded him that she did not write very well and could only print but she was willing to try.

Then it was almost as if Miss Dailey whispered in his ear "You teach her to write, James". He stood up, punched his fist in the air and said quietly, "I will teach you. Come on, I have a special set of cards."

Consider your competency today as an adult in the three historical essentials of education Reading, Writing and Arithmetic. Which is the least difficult for you today? Now, try to imagine yourself sitting at your desk in your fourth grade classroom . Which of these three R,s was the most difficult for you then? Is it the same as now? Draw some conclusions and why they may have occurred.

Chapter 13

The Club

The new principal in James' first school had done his graduate work in cognitive science and had a special interest in handwriting, not just as an art, but as a science. When Dr. Blake heard about the after- school Handwriting Club he called Miss Dailey and Miss Finch to his office. "Why is this club after school? I would like to reintroduce the teaching of handwriting in kindergarten through fourth grade for all students. I think we will see reading and composition scores increase, as well as a deeper understanding of mathematics. Let's find a curriculum we could use."

The two teacher friends replied in unison, "I think we have already found one!" The adventure began in earnest. James was called in as an advisor based upon his experience. Luckily he still had his top hat and pointer! It was going to be his special privilege to introduce the cursive alphabet in his most theatrical performance to each of the classes in grades K-4 after the new school year began. Even better, he would receive extra points in middle school for his volunteer service.

Dr Blake approached Miss Dailey and Miss Wren to ask if they would be willing to serve as resource teachers for the mandatory

30 minute instructional block that would be beginning in grades K-4 in September. A chalkboard was to be installed in each room to allow students to stand for their handwriting exercises.

Standing before a board had been shown to develop both the vestibular (balance) and proprioceptive (awareness of position in space) systems, needed skills in this sedentary environment called school. Additionally the resistance from the chalkboard promotes deeper memory tissue. Both motor and impulse control provide the basis for good handwriting. Dr Rosa Hagin, working at Bellevue Medical Center, collaborated with Dr. Kephart, an early pioneer in the field of learning disabilities. Their studies concluded that reading, writing, language arts, comprehension and spelling could not be separated but formed a fundamental whole (personal discussion with Dr. Rosa Hagin 2005).

For decades, American students have begun their writing careers in first grade with the use of a "ball and stick" and its many variations. Historically, somewhere between second and fourth grades the magical moment is supposed to occur when they finally learn "adult writing," e.g. cursive. Some like it , others don't. By junior high most teachers no longer care which system students use and cursive often goes by the wayside in lieu of the system mastered first, manuscript. Let's take a glance back...

Manuscript was initially devised as a mechanical labeling system for printing and identifying medicines primarily because of its clarity and legibility. Then came a method called Chancery Cursive you might still see in your computer font options. Turns out that was Charlemagne's idea. It was a more proper way to send correspondence to friends.

In America In the early 1900's, Margaret Wise developed a modified italic font that would easily fit the strokes of the fountain pens used at that time (does that take you back to finger stains?)

Then Horace Mann established a highly influential school in which a cursive style became accepted nationally. By 1936 a standard model of cursive writing had become the norm. Print would be taught first, in all American schools, then around grade three, cursive would be introduced to the joy of some students, the agony of others. (Hanna, 1998)

According to the scholars of that day, manuscript was generally noted for its original function, labeling. Each letter was drawn stroke by stroke, words formed letter by letter. The writer's thoughts were fragmented by constant pen lifts and directional shifts. Cursive, in comparison, was designed for communication. Its fluidity matched the flow of thought necessary to communicate. Each word was a complete unit formed by one line in a continuous, rhythmic movement. The multi sensory combination of reading, spelling and handwriting was identified by Early and Nelson (1976) as one of the most significant benefits of cursive writing.

Take just a moment and locate a copy of either the Declaration of Independence or the Preamble to the Constitution. It seems our forefathers were superb thinkers and writers. Has it occurred to us that our children may not be able to read these documents?

Chapter 14

The Summit

Miss Dailey had spent the day becoming re-acquainted with her own abilities to write in cursive. She too had defaulted to print. It did not take long to rediscover this fine gift (she was now beginning to see it as that). Both teachers felt as though they were about to take the ride of their lives. A singular joy came over them as they realized the far-reaching implications for such an assignment. They met again at their favorite coffee shop to explore the fresh landscape. This time they asked James to join them. After an invigorating discussion, they decided on an appropriate motto for this new adventure into inner space.

How can I know what I think until I see what I say?

E. M Forester

Scientists concur that skilled writing is one of the most demanding of all cognitive activities. The brain handles one continual task at a time. In order for the focused task to be clear, accurate sentences, both handwriting and spelling must become automatic skills. Writing is a visual activity guided by the writer's eyes but also a spatial activity as it applies to organizing text. In young writers, difficulties of composing text are related to high demands involved in the process of producing legible, accurate words. (Graham and Harris, 2000)

The ability to write automatically, without thinking of how to form the letters, frees the writer to consider what to say rather than how the letters are supposed to look. Although writing is still widely seen as a central aim of schooling, many students never learn to write with flexibility and skill.

Vocabulary knowledge, sentence structure and spelling need time and practice to develop over grade levels. Luria said the kinetic melody involved in writing words with a pen or pencil may play a role in learning how to spell them. This process does not transfer in the same way from a keyboard. (Handwriting Summit Washington, DC, 2010)

Miss Dailey and Miss Wren had gathered their data and a grand plan was beginning to form. The necessary chalkboards were ordered for grades K-4. These pioneering teachers tried them out. They were surprised to find that it was not as easy as they thought. Holding the chalk with the correct grip made the elbow unmanageable. Their feet shuffled, the opposite arm moved strangely. It was awkward trying to keep the chalk silent.... and the chalk dust..."Oh, my", both warbled in unison. Let's call James.

Personal Reflection

Think about how you felt about writing on a chalkboard when you were in elementary school. Did you ever have eraser cleaning duty? Did you ever draw a hopscotch design on the sidewalk with chalk? Spend a few minutes thinking about what we have traded for these experiences in today's culture. If you have young children or grandchildren, get a pack of jumbo chalk sticks and let them draw on the sidewalk or driveway. It will be a stimulating activity preparing their brains to write.

Chapter 15

Glancing Back in Time

The Lost World of Colonial handwriting

The ability to read in the newly founded America was treasured largely as the means to gain direct access to Scripture. Reading was taught first, writing second. The novice writer learned to cut a proper nib from a goose, raven or crow quill with a penknife. The execution of handwriting required no small degree of dexterity or skill." (Thornton, p.15) Copybooks began to circulate among the pioneers . Penmanship self instruction manuals emerged because it was considered that those that can "Reade may Learne to Write of themselves. (Thornton, p.5).

One colonist expressed with some chagrin that she could "Read readin' but could not read writin'. Many could read but not write. Well-bred women in early America kept private journals. For women, the ability to write in a clear hand was a relic from the old country and depended solely on breeding. At some point the clergy in Colonial America developed a need to write sermon notes, physicians found the need to write prescriptions and business men desired to keep ledgers. It was said that "Whoever

would be a man of business must be a man of correspondence."
(Watts, 1716).

Yet many wrote in an untrained hand. Indeed, writing at this
early stage of colonial life was not considered one of the three
R's of schooling. Then, in the new and developing America there
arose a new kind of school and a new kind of teacher, a "Writing
Master". Many of these gentlemen had no more than 30 hours of
writing instruction themselves but they saw an opportunity and
opened up schools announcing their services on a billboard. One
such entrepreneur "worked up a system" in which he had 115
scholars and his fame began to rise." (Thornton, p45)

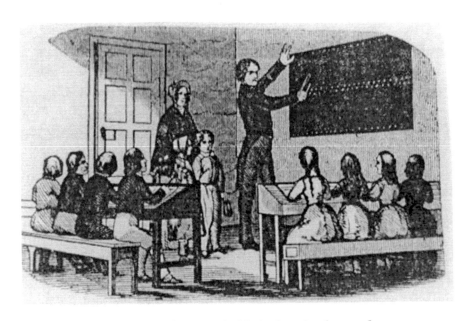

The separation of boys and girls in the schoolroom, from a
mid-nineteenth-century copybook.

It was not long before colonial schools were formed and
handwriting began to be considered as an important element in
the education of children. However, boys were to be trained in a

different kind of hand than girls. Boys learned a fast and legible script, suitable for business and public affairs while girls were taught in a smaller "hand" suitable for social skills, letter writing and calling card etiquette. The preference of training leaned heavily toward boys writing, girls sewing.

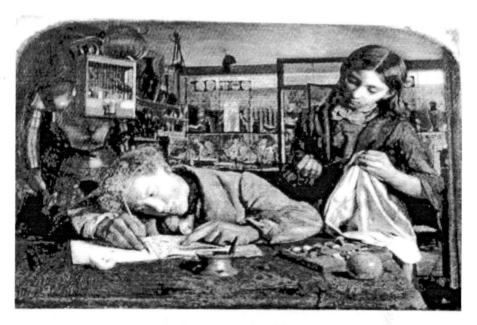

The boy writes, the girl sews.

As America moved into the Victorian age an interesting device was invented to encourage freedom in penmanship, the "talantograph. It was believed that a "poor hand" betrayed an ill-formed mind and smacked of vulgarity and negligence. Handwriting, they believed, revealed character. Muscles, then, must be under control of the will. This new device was designed to promote whole arm movement, clear handwriting and a more noble character. For clear handwriting, in the mind of our forefathers, elevated character, built inner discipline and revealed a cultivated taste as well as a disciplined imagination.

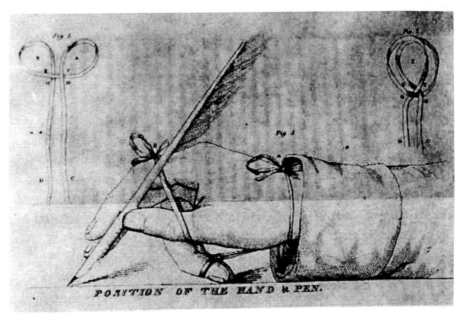

POSITION OF THE HAND & PEN.

The talantograph, a Victorian device to encourage "freedom" in penmanship.

Soon America's schools began incorporating the reading of Scripture with the writing of it by copying and thereby more easily memorizing the texts. A mid nineteenth century copybook contained this picture of a schoolmaster directing a handwriting lesson in a typical school of the day where boys and girls were separated. Masterful sweeping movements of the arms were emphasized affirming the manliness of penmanship, or command of the hand. Interestingly, handwriting became masculine domain in the colonial era for the main uses for handwriting were mercantile and commerce was a man's world. Men also, it was believed, were prey to base, physical appetites. The physical act of writing demanded direct decision and masterly effort, thereby overcoming these tendencies. (Thornton)

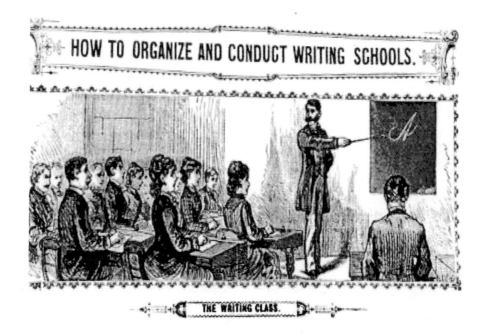

A Gilded Age itinerant writing school for ladies and gentlemen.

Then, along came the printing press. Did script become obsolete with this new invention? Interestingly, the Gutenberg invention did not appear in the American colonies until 1639 where it was established in the Massachusetts Bay Colony. Throughout the whole of the 17th century only five presses found their way to the colonies. The main reason for these new devices for the American consumer was to print religious books. What characterized the medium of print was above all its impersonality. Print lost any association with the hand just as pointedly as script retained it. (p, 29, Thornton). "What defined printing, then and distinguished it from handwriting was…its negative relation to the hand."(Thornton, p. 28). Letters of the alphabet had been creatively formed into human figures to try to contrast the impersonality of typeset letters. This 17th century human alphabet captures the preference of hand written calligraphy as opposed to machine driven print. Copies of these letters can still be seen in Colonial Williamsburg.

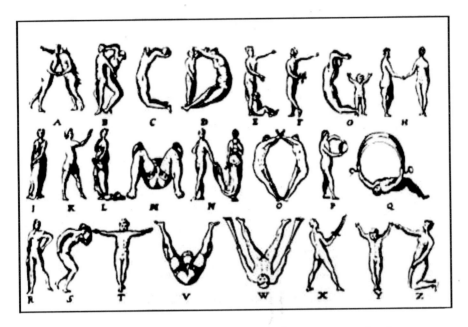

A human alphabet, from a seventeenth-century copybook.

Fast forward to the late 1800's when penmanship began to be considered a marvelous physiological habit that could be trained and then embedded in the mind so that it need not be continually brought to the surface of conscious thought leaving room to think about what to write rather than just how. A sketch of this process was circulated among the scientific community. Indeed, motor learning was being described.

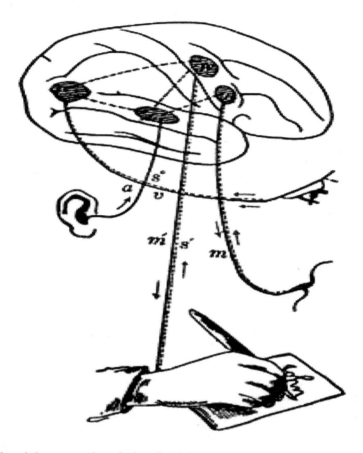

Handwriting as physiological habit, from William James,
Principles of Psychology, 1890.

The new knowledge paved the way for the Spencerian and Palmer
methods which found their way into progressive schools.
Learning to write, they explained, involved developing efficient
neural pathways to the appropriate muscles." (Thornton, p.146).
So another device appeared to guide correct movement of the
hand. This one appears somewhat tortuous particularly in light

of the belief in the early 1900's that left handers should be taught to write with their right hands. There was to be a certain rhythm in the writing, not to a metronome, as was an earlier tool, but the acquisition of an inner sense of movement.

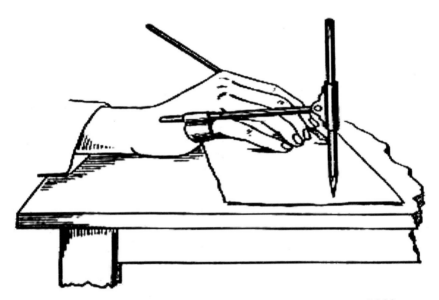

Laboratory analysis of the handwriting movement, 1903.

New ideas were generated in 1912 that acknowledged the mechanical constraints of young children coordinating pen and ink as well as the need for precise movements on lined paper. Learning to write, therefore, would be better done at a chalkboard. The teacher would call out the rhythm for each letter. Students were encouraged to develop their individual style once the basics of form had been mastered.

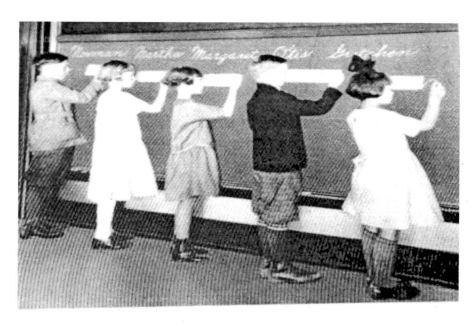

Practicing Palmerian push-pulls, 1912.

Palmer, whose writing methods were widely used in schools, stressed movement over form and placed emphasis on drill and practice. This, he believed was the method of implanting unconscious muscular habits, rather like learning to play the piano. Many attacked him as an amateur. However, as the handwriting discipline found its way into our nation's schools they began to reflect a strong cultural coherence.   (Thornton, 1996)

The Palmer drills seemed to please many children who reported to "love practicing their penmanship". (Thornton, p162). It also seemed to have a powerful effect on immigrant children imparting among other things, a physical grace where once there was "only coarseness" (Thornton, p.162) The day of the copy book was gone. Through this new penmanship the dominant thought was to "swing along fast! in perfect harmony with the spirit of the age, that of fast progress. (Thornton). Penmanship calisthenics were part of the school day.

Even more telling, teachers at the turn of the century vowed that within a decade (1900-1910) the problem of illiteracy would be erased. They believed they had the right tools formed within their intensive education in Teacher's Colleges. This impressive knowledge focused on the three strand cord of reading, writing and spelling (what scientists today call the "literacy braid).

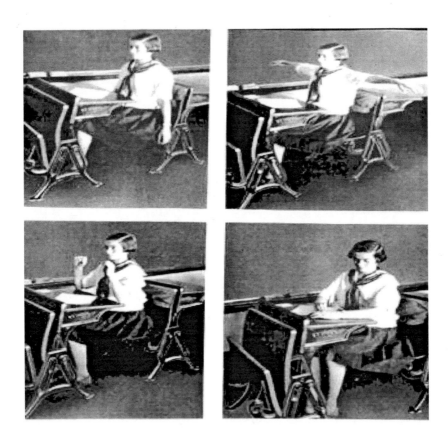

Penmanship Calisthenics 1924.

As business and commerce widened in America the typewriter threatened to "boot out" cursive writing. Many bemoaned its passing. It seemed that a transition to type removed all personal creativity or, more specifically human diversity in form and function. At the same time the penmanship pedagogues were facing down the machine due to its impersonal nature. Adults remembered fondly their days of pen and ink instruction and wanted it for their children.These were the days when moral certainty still seemed possible.

Interestingly, in 1899, Edward Johnston, the leader of a calligraphy revival ,was a Quaker of some wealth and social status. He was a graduate from the University of Edinburgh who had begun to study historic manuscripts in England. The root of his discontent with the current trend away from handwriting was the "soullessness" of modernity and the human alienation engendered by the machine. (p. 179 Thornton).

Johnston affirmed the dominance of the hand over the pen so as to control it to make the desired letters. The cry was heard, "Rejoice in humanness! Machines can't make mistakes." (Thornton, p182)

What horrified most observers of the penmanship decline in post war America was not so much its lack of individuality but its illegibility. "It was the Depression decade that was cited as the last decade of quality handwriting".(Thornton, p 184). Indeed, executives had secret codes of their own. We became a nation of "scrawlers". Teachers' colleges no longer trained teachers in the techniques of penmanship. When novice teachers entered the classroom they taught their students how to print and the transition to cursive was never accomplished satisfactorily . Poor handwriting has caused the nation's businesses big money. In

1955 the estimate was $70,000,000 a year through illegible inventory lists, **address labels,** etc. translating to economic inefficiency that continues today.

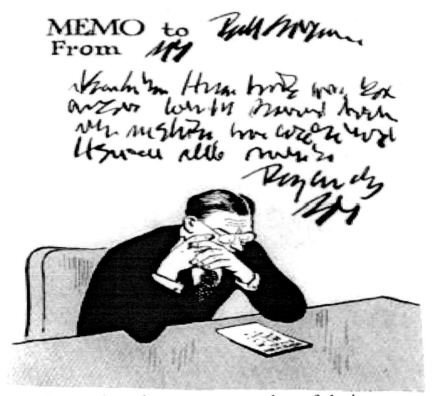

Executives have secret codes of their own.
A lighthearted penmanship jeremiad from the 1950's

How Far We Have Fallen

These students are in 5th grade assigned to special education classes, just as James was. They are at a strategic point in their lives in which literacy matters. Who can help them? Is it too late? We have the knowledge. Let's build the tools.

Student Scans

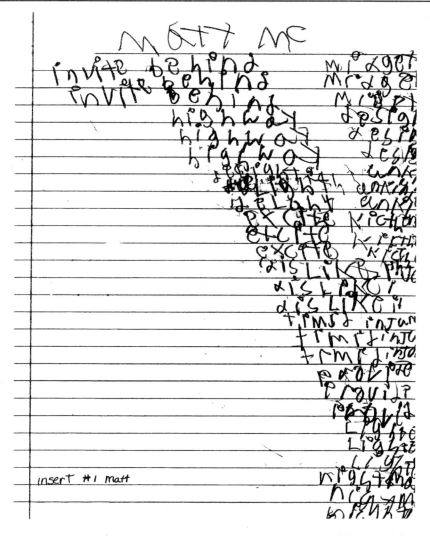

insert #1 matt

The pain of writing is evident here. I can imagine the student leaning farther and farther down his arm on the desk and murmuring, "what are these words anyway?"

3x Each

√ Great job!

1. invite	invite	invite
nightmare	nightmare	nightmare
2. lighten	lighten	lighten
unkind	unkind	unkind
3. provide	provide	provide
timid	timid	timid
behind	behind	behind
childish	childish	childish
highway	highway	highway
dislike	dislike	dislike
midget	midget	midget
injured	injured	injured
excite	excite	excite
kitchen	kitchen	

Well, this time the lines seemed to help. "My teacher thought it was good but I actually cannot read my own writing."

10 - 16 - 15

If i colo go to l.
concarl in the vild I
go t l elil becas: J
the Seninx, & the f
ar amezinl. I Like
Trees, And caves.
and it also has
crysis agrint,
to explor tourd
sac
are net, sanc
hav the oligins
beds and mives.
r ile river is
mqa water sous
promss are rly
so know you know
the cunsul iwl.
vizit

Halfway through this one I forgot what I was supposed to be saying and this does not look like the words I meant to say.

10/16/15

If I could visit any country in the world I would like to go to Irlin because my mom is going on Halloween my mom is flying out to Boston on Hallou then she and my papa and uncol pal then the next Day I wanted to go but I have school but allso it wose My moms gragwayshune gift from nersing drarey. So now you know were I lik to go.

This work is nearly legible when the student defaulted to print. I think the country to be visited is Ireland. There is little regard for correct spelling, however. How does a teacher grade this?

.√1 On Tuesday I hard tar wa:
forest fire.
√2 Youngest is the oposi from o
3 I so a kind lok at my pape
mow he was a cheater.
4 Westrday a lot of voters c
to vote.
5 A cleaner is a prsin how cle
home's. like a made,

This is another painful example of a bright mind yearning to be free. He is casually trying to respond to five questions. A check mark is given.

Devlin   10/19/15   '7

Once upon a time there
was a pack of deer. One day
they vent out they go out
to abreg a man vas they
git away from here house
then they dad depresd
wey ther yer intumn im tre
thdeyin so leve okjed
thder but we want come bac
then thay left

**What must a teacher do with this? Many would respond,
"Put him on a computer. I wonder if that would really help?
See the translation below.**

Devlin

Once upon a time there was a pack of deer. One day they went for a walk. While they were about to go over the bridge a man appeared. Don't go further. Why asked the male deer. I am the guardian of the bridge. So the deer left and did not return. Well not exactly...

This student has great ideas that ought to be able to flow from his pencil to a paper, effortlessly.

Jul ⑧ 1/2 1/6

jack when't to the store
to get a jacket. and the jalks
were on a rack.

The class was makeing
a paper snow man. They
mand 3 clecisls and put
on the dresous. Then
they put tele stick on
it they hed to stick it
on it was sticky

This attempt looks truly painful. There are smudges, signs of frustration, some good vocabulary trying to emerge. I wonder when he/she will just stop trying?

I ~~will~~ run up the _hill_
to go to my houns then I
will go insted and get a
dreenk, when I was poring
it I mad a ~~small~~ _spill_
so I ~~called~~ my mom to
get a partawol.

The uncertainty of what to say is controlling vocabulary usage. Really, what is he trying to say?

2/10/16

Who lost there tooth and cryed yesterday a-12:00 by Pulling the tooth out?

Who brock the brick yesterday at 1:10 becau they where made?

how did You print out the pictere yesterday?

The pain of putting down what could be very coherent thoughts never quite made it to the paper. For an 11 year old, this will only become worse.

if I had a magic pebble I
would wish for wings because
it would be fun to fly
with the berds and my
wings would be gour and
thall shimer and shine
and you can see them
a millie away the clods
will Be riiy flusy and
Soft the watr will gilmer
as I go I cod see avery.
thing and pepll will look
like ants.

There is a certain legibility here that demonstrates some
motor control, but observe the spelling and punctuation
errors. At age 12, written expression will continue a
downward spiral.

1-21-16

I. have at nitge herd
a story abot a Boy who shal
Choke on a petch.

When ever I go to school
I plop on my char.
In the morning I Broke
mom's faverit vase when
I Played Ball in the howse.
The patyoe was made
of stone.

**Free writing seems to have no rules. It seems the lesson
was just to" write your thoughts". Because it is
decipherable, there would most likely be no penalties.**

If I had a magin pappl
If I had a magic pebble
I whod wish for a Pand because
thay are big and Flaffy and cdoly.
And if I had to cwish for
a hodoher thing it whod be
a pappl. Because thay are
veay small and cute.

**The concept of what one would do with a "magic pebble"
seems quite lost in both the physical and mental pressure
of putting pen to paper.**

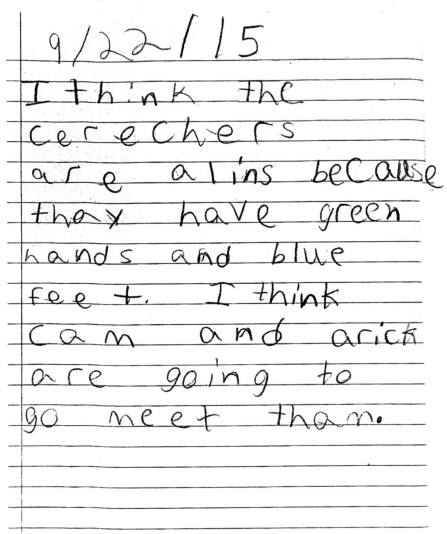

9/22/15

I think the cerechers are alins because thay have green hands and blue feet. I think Cam and arick are going to go meet tham.

The complexity of putting simple ideas on paper depends much upon the physical act of writing to be "hard-wired". When one must think both how to make the letters and then what to say, clear expression is lost in the process. Where is the content?

10-22-15

I saw a Dctor readmit he Pashont.

I refilld my glas with millk.

Wen the post war was over the sogers rejost.

Here there are some prompts that need a response. At age 12 the doubling rule works for both "refilld" and "millk". This is a student with good vocabulary skills as the last sentence reads "When the post war was over the soldiers rejoiced. He is begging for help.

If I hade a magic pebble I would wish for a horse because I love horses and ride horses but they are a lot of work because you have to take care of them buy hay buy a satol pade and a satol a gerth and a wipe.

One sentence does it here; we do not need to worry about punctuation or spelling.

If I had a magic pebble I
would wish for all the lagos
the wold because lagos are m
toys to play with itotsowe I
allso wish that my mom and
dad won the lotery becaus
my mom and dad all ways
to wen the lotery the
1,000,000,000,000 trelyon lot

**There is some humor in this effort but also pathos. At age
11 will he soon tire of these attempts to communicate?**

Name: _____   Date: 12/22/15

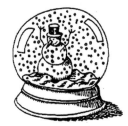

If I Was In a Snow Globe

Once apon a time I got a Snow globe for mom. She Love show globes. I got it at a spocy store that had a Lot of snow globes. There was a ladyd at the store and she look nice. So I foued the prefct one. It had Merry chimas it was chismint at the time.

So I got it and I cetaely droped it in the Lacks Face. She stared at it for a secdents. Then she plcd out a word and slad IN The porwer of the moon I slol prsh you.. I got trp ta in Not the snow globe that I got but diffent grat

There appear to be some coherent thoughts in this worksheet activity. The teacher needs to decide how to grade it. Teaching handwriting would have eliminated these errors.

MY   life   ends   in   a   snow   globe. It's
Wierd that the false   snow   mand me clood. Good
thing I had a coat. I had a coat because it was
snowing out side and   it was clan and un—
comtherdel.

there was   a snow man in there   and that
talked. So I said hi and he frozed. I saw
a axc on a tadl and   I thot That
I code get the ax c and breah the
glass. The snow man seid he can help.
I toed him I need to get out and
the and the vold stree.

we   got the axe a breh trow. The Snow
man help me brak trew because it was
the red to brake. So I said bye to thir
snow man, time to wrak up he No it
is just a drem. Now you Now what it
feel Like in a snow globe

This student is ready to move into middle school where the stakes are much higher. Chances are, all work will transfer to a keyboard and poor spelling will not be an issue. Will he enjoy reading and writing?

Name_____Devlin_____

Read each story carefully. Then follow the directions below.

Splish, Splash! Who Needs a Bath?

When Abbey got home from school, she went into the kitchen for a snack. In the kitchen, she saw muddy footprints on the floor and along the edge of the counter where the roast was cooking in the crock pot. She got the mop and bucket out of the pantry and cleaned up the footprints. Then she began looking for the dog to give him a bath.

1. Underline the words in the story that tell you why Abbey went into the kitchen. Circle the word that tells you where Abbey had been.

2. Why do you think Abbey wanted to give the dog a bath?
    _____Muddy Foot prints made her know the_____

3. How can you tell that Abbey has helped out with household chores before?
    _____She wold have givin the dog a bath_____
    _____befor_____

Home Sweet Home

Tony got home from spending the weekend away. He was just in time to wash up for dinner. He headed straight upstairs to the bathroom. He met his mom in the upstairs hallway carrying a load of laundry. He thanked her for fixing his favorite dinner, spaghetti and garlic bread. Then he said it sure would be good to sleep in his nice, comfortable bed after sleeping on that hard ground.

4. Underline the words in the story that tell you Tony knows it's just about dinner time. Circle the word that lets you know how long Tony had been gone.

5. How did Tony know what was for dinner? _____He Knew iF_____
    _____he was away he wold get a wish in_____

6. Why do you think Tony had been sleeping on the ground?
    _____Thee reni he went to wod on hike pay ba_____

Bonus: Write a short paragraph telling about a time you went camping or spent the night away from home. Use complete sentences.

Despite this worksheet structure the student's responses are barely legible. Early handwriting training would have set him free. Where is James now with his Handwriting Club?

Handwriting In America

I feel that Handwriting & Cursive writing need to be a core technique to learn in general. When I was growing up, I didn't do much learning on either subject. But I do know how to write in cursive. My handwriting isn't at its best but that means I am ready for improvement. Back when I was a first grader, I didn't like to write at all and I never got pushed to do it. Now it's getting better everyday because I don't want my handwriting to be sloppy.

Now I am 18 years old, and I feel that schools around the country need to do something about this travisty. Technology has taken over our brains, so we dont have to worry about writing correctly. It corrects it for us and that is so sad. We should steer away from technology and make the impossible possible. If we can do that, then we might be able to try to make Handwriting the best learning experience for everyone

Epilogue

The story about James is fictional. The pages of student writing are real. James is a prototype based upon the many students the author has known. It's purpose is to expose a problem needing to be addressed in our schools today. It may be the proverbial elephant on the table. The look back in our nation's belief in the power of writing is well-documented by scholars. Perhaps it is not too late for innovators in the field of education to sound an alarm. Technology will continue to evolve and our children will continue to be enamored by it. At what cost? We who love learning must respect the past as well as the vision for the future, giving a firm nod to all that technology can provide. Keyboarding is a fine tool for ease of writing once clear competence is established in spelling, reading and writing by hand. We stand to lose a great deal if we allow technology to become our master.

References

Berninger, V. *Evidence-Based, Developmentally Appropriate Writing Skills K-5: Teaching the Orthographic Loop of Working Memory to Write Letters, Spell Words, and Express Ideas.* University of Washington, Handwriting in the 21st Century: An Educational Summit, Washington, D.C., 2012

Bounds, G., Indiana University, *How Handwriting Trains the Brain,* WSJ, 2011.

Conti, D. *Kinematic and Clinical Correlates of Handwriting in Elementary School* Director Human Movement Laboratory, Wayne State University, 2012

Deardorff, J. *The Many Healthy Perks of Good Handwriting. The Virginian Pilot, 2011*

Datchuck, S. *Teaching Handwriting to Elementary Students with Learning Disabilities*: A *Problem Solving Approac*h, Teaching Exceptional Children, 2015

Early & Nelson. Indiana State University *The Case for Cursive Writing,* 1976

Grigorenko, E. *Writing: A Mosaic of New Perspectives.* Handwriting Summit, Washington, D. C. 2012

Hagin, R, Search and Teach. Walker Publishing. 1976

Hanna, J. 1998 *Does it Make a Difference?* National Institute for Learning Disabilities (NILD) Discoveries Spring, 1998

Hensher The Missing Link. The Lost Art of the Handwritten Note. WSJ, 2012

Hoag, C. *Schools try to stop trend that's erasing cursive writing* Associated Press, 2012

Hopkins, K. *Teaching How to Learn in a What to Learn Culture.* Jossey-Bass, 2010

Konnikova, M. New York Times *The Right Stuff,* 2014

la Cour, I*The Girl,* Academic Therapy. 1980

la Cour, I. *Cursive Writing as a Means to Read.* Academic Therapy. 1980

Mangen, A. & Velay, J. *Digitizing literacy: Reflections on the Haptics of Writing.* The National Centre for Reading and Education Research. University of Stavanger, Norway. Mediterranean Institute for Cognitive Neuroscience. Marseille, France 2008

Marr, D. & Windsor, M. *Handwriting Readiness: Locatives and Visuomotor Skills in the Kindergarten Year.* Utika College of Syracuse University. 2005

Orton, S. / Gillingham, A.

Peverly, S. *The Relationship of Transcription Speed and Other Cognitive Variables to Note-Taking and Test Performance.* Handwriting Summit, Washington, D.C. 2012

Rose, R *The Writing/Reading Connection.* 2004

Sortino, D. *Intelligence and the Art of Cursive Writing.* Educational Strategies. 2011

Technology and the Death of Handwriting, BBC News, 2008

The Many Healthy Perks of Good Handwriting. Virginian Pilot. 2011

Their Signatures Were Liberating, Independence Day, Virginians. Virginian Pilot. 2015

Thornton, T. *Handwriting in America:A Cultural History.* Yale University Press, 1996

Why Does Writing Make us Smarter? Huffington Post AOL

Zimmerman, D. National Institute for Learning Development. 1976